A Guide to Wellbeing After Stillbirth or Miscarriage

A Guide to Wellbeing After Stillbirth or Miscarriage

Book and Journal

Martina Simpson

SUNESIS MINISTRIES LTD

Published by Sunesis Ministries Ltd. For more information about Sunesis Ministries Ltd, please visit:

www.stuartpattico.com

ISBN: 978-1-9163874-1-6

Contents

Introduction

Angel Wings Gifts firstly would like to say sorry for the loss of your baby or babies and hope that this gift helps, as you channel the many different stages of your grief.

You may have received this gift from a loved one or hospital, or maybe even bought it for yourself. But the aim of this gift is to help you with some of the stages of grief that you may experience in this time, by giving you some tips as to how to cope with everyday life and the loss of your baby.

There will be some stories from other parents who have experienced baby loss via miscarriage or stillbirth, within this book. There is a Journal at the back of this book so that you can journal any thoughts and feelings you may be feeling and you may like to write a letter to baby. So be kind to yourself and take your time.

1

My Reason for Angel Wings

Hi, my name is Martina and I lost a baby in 2014 via miscarriage at twelve weeks. I was not planning to have a child at this time, as I was on contraception, the copper coil. However, I did get pregnant. Once I found out at six weeks, I went to the doctors and told them. To their amazement after a pregnancy test, they then removed the coil and told me to go to the early pregnancy ward weekly to get scanned. At this stage they could not measure a heartbeat, so they would measure the baby weekly up until the twelve-week mark to see if the baby was growing, which at this point would mean that the pregnancy would be safe to continue as normal.

So, week after week the baby continued to grow and even though I was advised by midwives not to get too attached until the twelfth week, the weekly positive scans naturally built anticipation of a new baby. Unfortunately, the day before my final weekly scan, at twelve weeks, I spotted a little blood. I had called my midwife, but she advised that sometimes that does happen, and recommended that I go to the scan the next day to find out.

When I arrived for the scan, they measured the baby and then brought me along with my husband into a room. They told me that the baby had not grown and that it seemed as if I had miscarried. I went instantly numb as I was being advised of my options. I had two options, either to remove the baby surgically the next day or let it miscarry naturally. The radiographer advised me to go for a coffee to think about it.

As I walked to the canteen, I felt numb. Even though I knew that I should not have become attached, based on the advice given at the beginning of the pregnancy, any woman who has become pregnant knows that instantly there is a bond that is uncontrollable. Since I did not have many words to say, my husband thought it was best to allow for a natural miscarriage, as the midwife did use words such as, "it would seem that you have miscarried". So, in his mind, we could be terminating a baby that just did not grow in the space of six days. I agreed and we went back downstairs.

The room was occupied when we returned, and the midwife was standing outside the door of the occupied room. She asked me in front of all the people waiting in the waiting room, "So what have you decided?" I was enraged by the lack of care of this sensitive issue as I watched women stare at me, hearing her ask me this question. As I was so numb and stunned by her lack of care I said, "Naturally". She replied, "Great I will put that on your notes. Take care. Bye". And she walked off.

I left the hospital with loss of all feeling, enraged, angry and hurt by this experience. I spent just over a month in a state of depression, but knew I needed to pull myself out of it. So, as no-one around me really knew what to do I 'googled' and found a website dealing with how to get over grief of losing a baby. All this time I had not cried once, and knew that would help me to find release. I eventually found my release and got the help I needed.

However, it always stuck with me that women who experience baby loss, either through miscarriage or stillbirth are just meant to dust themselves off and get on with life. This then brought to my attention, women who had experienced stillbirth and had to deliver their baby. When having conversations with other women who have lost babies, they all say the same statements: -

"Baby loss is a taboo but yet happens to so many women".

Hearing these sentiments led me to this idea of gift boxes for women who have items that help them to put themselves first, and in addition, a book that could help them to channel through the stages of grief and give them comfort. This book is compiled of lots of women's experiences, with testimonials and information to help you through this time.

2

Stages of Grief

Grief, as a general subject, is a very individual experience and there is no exact science of the way it plays out in your life. The emotional impact of grief is sometimes felt instantly after a stillbirth or miscarriage. However, sometimes it can take some time. It is common to feel tired, lose your appetite and have difficulty sleeping after a miscarriage or stillbirth. You may also feel a sense of guilt, shock, sadness and anger – sometimes at a partner, or at friends or family members and from those who have had successful pregnancies.

People grieve in different ways. Some find it comforting to talk about their feelings, while others find the subject too painful to discuss. When speaking to counsellors, many of them use the Ross and Kessler (2005) approach which posits that there are five stages of grief, which are detailed below. Even though 'grief' is a generic term, for the purposes of this journal, I have personalised it to the loss of a baby:

Denial: Life makes no sense. You will feel in a state of shock and denial and numb. You wonder how you can go on, if you can go on, why you should go on. Denial and shock help us to cope and make survival possible. Denial helps us to pace our feelings of losing our baby. There is a grace that comes with denial. It is nature's way of letting in only as much as we can handle at the time. As you accept the reality of the loss and start to ask yourself questions, you are beginning the healing process. You are becoming stronger, and the denial is beginning to fade. But as you proceed, all the feelings you were denying begin to come up again for you.

Anger is a necessary stage of the healing process. We usually know more about suppressing anger rather than expressing or feeling it. Look at your anger as an expression of the intensity of your love and protection for your baby. Be willing to feel your anger. The more you truly feel it, the more it will begin to dissipate and the more you will heal. Anger is the emotion we are most used to managing. The truth is that anger has no limits. It can extend not only to your friends, the doctors, your family, yourself and even your baby, but also to God. You may ask, "Why is God doing this to me?" Anger is strength, even though at times it can feel out of control, and it can be an anchor. Initially, losing your baby may feel like being lost at sea, with no connection to anything. Then you get angry at someone, maybe a person who did not attend the funeral, or maybe a person who isn't around. The anger becomes a bridge over the open sea, a connection from you to them.

Bargaining: Okay, truce. "What if I devote the rest of my life to helping others? Then can I wake up and realise this has all been a bad dream?" We become intertwined in moments of "If only..." or "What if..." statements. We want life returned to what it was. We ask ourselves, "Was it the burger I ate" or "Was it the way I slept"? Guilt is often a companion to bargaining. The "if onlys" cause us to find fault in ourselves and what we "think" we could have done differently. We may even bargain with the pain, trying to negotiate our way out of the hurt.

Depression: This depressive stage feels as though it will last forever. It is important to understand that this depression is not a sign of mental illness. It is the appropriate response to a great loss. We can withdraw from life, left in a thick cloud of intense sadness, wondering: *Is there any point in going on? Could this be the time to end my relationship with my partner?* If grief is a process of healing, then depression is one of the many necessary steps along the way.

Acceptance is often confused with the notion of being "all right" with what has happened. This is not the case. This stage is about accepting the reality that our baby is physically gone and recognising that this new reality is the permanent reality. As you may be reading this, you may not be ready to handle this stage just yet, and that is fine. This stage, however, does eventually come and we learn to accept it. In resisting this reality, at first many people want to maintain life as it was before losing the baby. In time, we see that we cannot maintain the past. It has been forever changed and we must adapt. Finding acceptance may be just having more good days than bad ones. As we begin to live again and enjoy our life, we may feel that in doing this, we are betraying our baby. We can never replace what has been lost, but we can make new and beautiful memories. Instead of denying our feelings, we listen to our needs; we change, we grow, and we evolve. We begin to live again, but we cannot do so until we have given grief its time.

George Engel (1959) states that... "the loss of a loved one is psychologically traumatic..." He compares being physically wounded the same as being psychologically wounded through a loss. Both need a period of time to bring the body and mind back to a balance.

These five stages detailed above, are not systematic. You can jump around these areas multiple times.

At the back of this book are some blank pages for you to journal your thoughts. It has been proven that journaling helps you to articulate how you are feeling. Questions that could help you start could be:

- *What stage of grief do you feel you are currently at and why?*
- *How do you feel about the people around you?*
- *How do you feel the people around you can help you?*

Give yourself time to be sad, frustrated and angry. Give yourself time to heal, accept, and to grow. Time does not erase anything, but it can provide you with enough space to be able to breathe again. And then one day you wake up and your heart is a little brighter.

3

Your Health and Wellbeing

Baby loss definitely is a time where you need to give more attention to yourself for a while. Sometimes the trauma of your loss may cause intrusive thoughts, flashbacks or nightmares. Below are some of the thoughts some have experienced:

- *I 'should' be coping better.*
- *I 'should' be stronger or be able to offer more support to my partner.*
- *It was my fault.*

Worrying a lot is exhausting. It can create negative thought patterns and change how you behave. It may also make it harder to focus on things that could help you feel better. Take one day at a time. It is okay to have these feelings of grief, anger, resentment and so much more. They will not always feel this strong.

Eating properly and looking after yourself are hugely important and below I have covered some areas for health and wellbeing. It is not unusual for bereaved parents, particularly mums, to become obsessed with their own, their partner's or their other children's health. Your own mortality can come to the forefront of your mind – if a tiny baby can die, so can anyone. This reaction usually fades with time.

GIVE YOURSELF TIME

Grief is a unique and personal thing for every individual and the best way for you to have healthy wellbeing is to take your time. Be attentive to how you are feeling and follow that through. Talk to people around you about how you are feeling, no matter how unpleasant it may sound.

If you are having a bad day, maybe focus on accomplishing one thing for the day. It may be washing your hair or going for a walk. But the main thing is that you give yourself time.

LET US TALK

For many women who have had a stillbirth or miscarriage, talking is the last thing on your mind, especially if you have to talk about how you are feeling. But it is essential. It helps not only those who are closest to you to understand how you are feeling, but it also releases you from any feelings that are bringing you discomfort. Many women say that talking has been one of the biggest healers for them as it helps them to not feel trapped by their own thoughts and also to channel through the stages of grief a little easier. Your partner is essentially one of the best to talk to as he/she will be in their own stage of grief and sometimes it is comforting to know that you are not alone. Some may find that they cannot go to anyone they know. For this, I would advise counselling as it is a good way to sometimes leave those concerns with someone else and they can give you tips on how to channel through your grief. Sometimes finding the right counsellor can be tricky. Make sure that you are comfortable with your counsellor and if not, then find another - you are not obliged to stay with them.

WHAT TO EAT

Eating may be the last thing on your mind, but it is necessary. For some, you might have family members who may help with this. But eating the right foods plays a big part in your mood. Eating a balanced meal and staying away from junk foods can actually help reduce the feelings of anxiety and depression. If you are struggling to eat and can only snack on a few things, try to grab snacks that will nourish your body, like nuts or fruit. If you have loved ones around you and they would like to help, get them to make a few dishes that you could put in the freezer. When you have a good day, try to make a bulk of nutritional meals to put in the freezer.

LET US MOVE

"Going for a brisk stroll could play an important role in fighting depression," BBC News has reported. As much as you may be feeling deflated, get up and go for a walk, or to the gym, a home work out, or a run. Exercise increases your heart rate, which pumps oxygen to the brain. This then releases hormones which

provide excellent growth of brain cells and a sense of feeling good. Some people have found that even when not feeling great, coming back after a run has allowed them to be able to cope with the day a little better.

ASK FOR HELP

Finding people who you trust is sometimes really important for you in this time. Below is a list of things you could ask relatives or friends to help with:

- Washing your clothes
- Ironing
- Cooking
- Cleaning
- Just being in the house
- Taking your other children for a few hours or overnight
- Listening
- Sorting the garden
- Taking the dog for a walk

SEX

When grieving the death of a baby, people's feelings can also be very complicated. It would be natural to associate sex with creating your baby and this can cause anxiety or even anger about having sex. Accept the way you are feeling towards having sex. Some people may not feel ready or able to have sex. Others may find that it is comforting or reassuring to have sex. Grief can also lead to a loss of sexual desire for some people. In most cases, you can also feel that your body has *"let you down"* and your self-esteem and self-worth are affected. There may be new scars and changes to your body that are magnified by your loss. So, take your time and communicate with your partner on how you are feeling about sex. Make sure you have followed the guidance of the doctor in terms of sexual activity, which in most cases, the advice is to wait at least six weeks. However, even though six weeks is the estimated time for healing, grief is still something that can take time, and sex may not be something that you want to do straight away after your healing, and that is fine.

"After losing my baby I remember my husband wanting to have sex and asking if we could. I was not ready but felt like I had to give him that, as I was so not really giving him any time, from the time of the loss of our baby, it was the worst sexual experience we had ever had, as I got upset, and it set us back. I am a strong believer in waiting until you are ready. I did not realise that grief could affect me sexually."

FEELING ANGRY

Many women feel they have failed as mothers. They feel responsible for what has happened because their bodies let them down. With time, some mums also feel guilty when they start to feel a little better, as if they are not honouring their baby or 'forgetting them'. Anger is a very natural part of grief. Many parents direct this towards the hospital, or towards friends and family. For some women it is a generalised anger at the injustice - *'Why me?'* All the feelings we mention here are normal.

Another hurdle is telling people who are close to you, which can be challenging as it can feel as if you have failed. This is dealt with in the next section.

4

How to tell people

There is no one right way to tell people about your loss. Remember that members of your family and close friends may have their own feelings about the news. You may even want to do it in different ways, depending on who you are telling. This also depends on how close they are and your relationship with that person. Whether you feel they will understand, or if they have experienced something similar. Note that they may be experiencing the loss too as they may have been looking forward to the birth of the baby; for example, becoming a grandparent.

Here are some examples of ways you could tell people:

- **Face to Face** – if you want hugs and emotional support and someone to listen to you, then this is a good way to tell someone whom you trust.
- **Friend** - another approach is to have someone else convey the news for you. Maybe your mum or sibling can call around and tell the rest of your family. Your manager or co-

worker could tell the people in your team or office. If there is something you would specifically want them to say or not say, then make that clear.

- **A thoughtful text or letter** - you might find it easier to write notes or send email messages to certain family members, friends, or co- workers. Explain briefly what happened and be honest about what you need in terms of support.

It may be of some shock to you, but people often have no idea what to say in the face of grief. Maybe they have never experienced a loss like this and truly cannot imagine what you are going through. Or they may be afraid they will say something to make it worse. Sometimes people just have a hard time handling grief or dealing with death. It may bring up their own feelings that they do not want to face. If you do not get a response, try to remember that people do care about you.

Some people may say things that actually make you feel worse. *"It will go better next time"* or *"I know how you feel"* may make you feel as though your grief is being swept under a carpet. Your loved ones do not mean to be insensitive. They may not understand that simply expressing something heartfelt like, *"I am so sorry about your stillbirth"* or *"I know how much you wanted this baby,"* is all they really need to say. Some may try to downplay your grief and, not everyone understands the impact of a pregnancy loss. As you go through this process, try to stay open. You may find you receive support from people and places you least expect.

Below are some questions to help you to work out how you would like to approach letting people know about your loss:

- What do I want people to know at work?
- How do I want to be treated on my return?
- Who do I want to tell – should I make a friends and family list?
- How do I want to tell my family?
- How do I want to tell my friends?
- What scares me about telling people?

5

Partners and children

It is often assumed when you lose a baby, that the mother is the main concern, partners are then expected to take on the supportive role. They tend to be the person who informs family and friends of your loss and sometimes end up running the home whilst the mother is recovering. The partner can be forgotten after a baby loss, as everyone looks to the mother to ease her load and cater to her emotionally. It is easy to overlook the fact that the partner and children need time and space to grieve too.

People grieve differently, everyone does not express their feelings outwardly. Some people find it difficult to express their emotions and their feelings can get locked up. This can be misinterpreted as lack of sympathy to the loss of their baby. It is not uncommon for the partners to take on the practicalities of life and keep themselves busy. It is important that you both make time to grieve in your own ways.

Sometimes if a person suppresses their grief it can display

itself randomly in a future moment, for example, if someone else has a baby, there can be a sudden feeling, if the grief has not been properly dealt with. Older siblings can deal with their grief differently, and may try to overcompensate for the baby who was lost. This is age related and of course, dependent on the understanding of the child. There are some very helpful bereavement books on the market for children to help them understand and comprehend their feelings. It can be important for the sibling to see parents grieving and have that explained to them. This can get them in touch with their own emotions too. If you see that your child is struggling with the grief of the baby loss, maybe talking to someone else could help. This could be someone who they are quite open to talking to, like a grandparent or aunt, as some children still will not want to bog their parents down with their feelings based on the situation.

Also, sometimes couples feel that because they lost a baby, together, they you must grieve together. We all deal with grief differently and there may be times when you need to be alone. Some couples found it easier to deal with their grief together, but if your partner is not inclined to do so, then do not push them as they may just be at a different stage to you. Give them time and let them know you are there if needed.

Below, I have identified some ways for partners and children, or even yourself, to connect to their grief and you could suggest these to them:

Yoga - Yoga is an ancient form of exercise that focuses on strength, flexibility and breathing to boost physical and mental wellbeing. The main components of yoga are postures. A few classes could really improve your wellbeing and focus.

Ask for help - when contacting people and letting them know the news, you could ask them to cook some meals and bring them over, or look after the children so you can have some down time; or do the ironing or simply ask for some space if you need it. This will allow you to connect with your grief.

Mindfulness - means knowing directly what is going on inside and outside ourselves, moment by moment. It is easy to stop noticing the world around us. It is also easy to lose touch with the way our bodies are feeling and to end up living 'in our heads' – caught up in our thoughts without stopping to notice how those thoughts are driving our emotions and behaviour. Mindfulness is also about reconnecting with our bodies and the sensations they experience. This means waking up to the sights, sounds, smells and tastes of the present moment. That might be something as simple as the feel of a banister as we walk upstairs. You can find mindfulness videos on YouTube which will help with your mental wellbeing.

Count to ten before reacting/responding – sometimes there may be comments made around you that may be insensitive and the best way to respond is to count and think about your response as you are channelling through grief.

Counselling – you may see that if your partner is not opening up, maybe speaking to a counsellor to voice all of your inner thoughts, without it getting to the people you love the most, could be helpful. Your partner may be in a state of anger or rage that they may not feel comfortable to express to you or friends and family.

Stress gadgets to squeeze – you will be surprised that sometimes the transference of stress from your hand to a stress gadget can be hugely impactful when you are feeling instantly overwhelmed.

Get involved in a sport/ run/ exercise – this will help to clear your head and release any tensions in the body.

Talk to their male/female friends – this, believe it or not, is the best time to talk to a good friend who simply wants to be able to do anything to help. If you just want a listening ear, friends can be perfect in this situation, and if you are not sure if they will interject with questions, maybe start by saying, "I just want you to listen".

Talk to each other – this will probably have a dual effect as you will be able to hear how your partner is feeling and you can also express how you are feeling about the loss of your baby. This technique works well because you both know the feelings you felt as you were planning for the arrival of him/her and you can be as raw as you need to be with each other as to where you both are and give each other support on the good and bad days.

Writing it down – start with how your day has been and then see where the pen takes you. We have had many testimonials where people have written more than they intended and ended up expressing elements of how they are feeling about the loss of their baby. This resulted in them finding comfort in seeing their what they are feeling set out on a page, rather than keeping them locked inside their heads.

Organisations - there are many organisations that offer

groups and free sessions to couples and families who need additional support. If you would like some additional support, then visit our website (www.angelwingsgifts.co.uk) where you will find a list of organisations that can help.

"I did not realise that I did not deal with my grief until we were considering to have another baby and then I felt an overwhelming feeling of anxiety. I started getting angry at my partner every time she tried to pick up something that was a little heavy, or sometimes even when she had finished in the toilet checking that she was smiling when she came out, because that meant she was not bleeding, I know crazy. But it helped me to talk to my partner about my anxiety and how I was feeling, and because she had dealt with her grief previously, she was able to help me through it." Leon

6

Returning to Work

For some parents, going back to work can feel daunting. For others, the routine of work can be helpful. Once you have agreed a date to return to work, you may find it helpful to talk to your manager or employer about how you are feeling and what might help you settle into the work environment. You could also ask to visit your workplace and meet up informally with your colleagues before you return to work. Think about how you might like to share the news with your manager or your colleagues and whether you would like to tell everyone directly, or have your manager or a trusted colleague tell people on your behalf. If you named your baby, you could share the name, anything you feel comfortable sharing about how baby died, and anything else you feel is relevant for them to understand. Let your employer know if there is anything you would like them to do or communicate to colleagues that you feel would be helpful for you.

Being back at work, in addition to settling into your role after a period of absence, there are various things which might feel difficult for you. There might be colleagues who are pregnant or those who visit during their maternity leave to introduce their new baby. There might also be colleagues who have experienced the death of a baby at an earlier time. If you are the birth mother, colleagues may have seen you pregnant so might be more sensitive to your situation. For fathers, co-mothers, adoptive parents and foster parents, the loss may seem less obvious to other people and more isolating for you. Grief can be tiring. You may be surprised at how exhausted you feel and you might find that you struggle to concentrate.

You may find that you are very sensitive to what people say, or that you lack confidence about making decisions. Some parents become frustrated with themselves and anxious that they can no longer cope with work. However, all of these reactions are common effects of grief and should pass with time and support. If you suddenly feel overwhelmed, take a break if you can. You could possibly go for a short walk or find a quiet space to be alone. You may also find it helpful to find somewhere private to talk to a colleague, phone a family member or friend. However, just take one day at a time. Use the journal in the back of this book to answer the questions posed below:

- How are you feeling about going back to work?
- Who are you most nervous about speaking to or seeing?
- What information do you want your colleagues to know and how do you want to be treated?

Revisit these questions before returning to work as feelings do change and you may want to change your responses.

7

Creating positive memories

With so little to remember your baby by, it can be difficult to know how to commemorate the huge loss of both, baby, and the future that might have been. Below I have collated some examples of ways that you could create a lasting memory for your baby:

Tribute - Whilst the grieving process often begins as private and intimate, some then choose to honour their baby's short life with a tribute page, in which donations are given to a charity of choice. This allows friends and family to show their support through messages and donations.

Memory box – it contains items that are related to the birth and that will, in future, allow you to remember your baby and this time, with more clarity. Some hospitals offer memory books for you to record details and measurements of your baby, scans, clothing that you had bought baby, letters you may have received, or letters that you may have written to baby, a lock of their hair. Many parents can end up getting quite creative and painting and decorating their box to best reflect their baby and family. You are also welcome to use *Angel Wings* gift box to use as your memory box.

Photo Album or picture frame - You may have had scanned pictures, or a picture of their hands or feet taken at the birth and you may wish to put those images up on your wall or in a family album. Some parents in the future end up showing a surviving child their sibling(s).

Bauble – As a family you might want to create a bauble to place on a tree or hang in your home in remembrance of baby.

Anniversaries – As time moves on, some parents decide to mark the day baby was born as the baby's birthday and celebrate that day, either by getting a helium balloon with the age they would be, and letting it off into the sky on the day of their birthday. Or, there may be other points within the year that may trigger a feeling of grief; this could be the due date, Mother's day, Father's day, Christmas, or the day of baby's funeral. These can be challenging days and so you may want to set aside time for you to reflect.

Jewellery – you may want to get a piece of jewellery engraved or a locket with a picture inside to always wear.

Plant a tree – some parents plant a tree in their garden or in a special place in memory of baby.

Funeral – if your baby was born after twenty-four weeks, you are required to bury or cremate your baby's body. This is a way to remember and can involve extended family and close friends if you would like.

You may feel at present that you are not ready to do any of the above, as the loss may be too much at this time. However, many parents have soon regretted the decision to get rid of all memories as life moves on and they come to terms with what has happened; keep them in a box for the time being whilst you are in this season. As time goes on, surges of grief may hit you occasionally and most of the time, will come to you unexpectedly and sometimes having these items and memories can help with the pain.

Be kind to yourself. Give yourself time and space to grieve and to remember your baby.

"On what would have been my Angel baby's eighteenth Birthday I held a fund-raising Gala and raised a considerable amount of money in celebration of his eighteenth and to a charity that helps other families that have lost babies. The night was amazing and marked his birthday in a beautiful way" Sandra

WRITE IT OUT. DANCE. BANG A DRUM. GET PAINT ALL OVER YOUR BODY. SING TILL YOU'RE BREATHLESS. BE LIKE A CHILD. CREATIVITY WILL UNLOCK IN BOTH HEALING AND HOPE.

8

Another Baby?

Some family members or friends during your grief, may suggest having another baby, as they may feel it could help. For some families, trying after a loss has been the best thing for them as they did not want to wait. However, some families decided to wait a while. The decision is completely yours and your partner's, so do not feel pressure either way. Some families decide not to have another at all because they could not deal with the idea of losing again. I think overall, be honest with yourselves and let time tell. You may well make a decision now to never have another child again and then in a year's time you may change your mind and be ready to try again, with the possibility of losing again, but mentally you will be in a better place.

If deciding to have another baby, discuss with your partner certain credentials, like, do you want to use the same hospital or midwife as before, or do you want to attend counselling throughout your pregnancy?

Planning for another baby may be difficult as you have experienced a loss already. Preparing a nursery, getting a new cot, or preparing a hospital bag may fill you with anxiety, but take your time, there is no rush. of course you would like to have as much ready for the baby as possible; but if all you have are a few clothes and a Moses basket, then if you have to ask grandparents or friends to get a few bits at the shops when the baby has come into the world, then that is fine also.

Some mothers feel like they are not building a strong enough bond with their baby in the pregnancy and are scared to overly bond in case they lose a baby again. This is normal, but if you feel this way then speak with someone.

"I can't try again, the idea of potentially losing another baby is not an option for me. I have been honest about my decision to not try again with my husband with also the idea that he may not want to continue a relationship with me not wanting to have a baby. He decided that he wanted to stay in our marriage. We are still together and still very much in love and happy". Audre

9

Getting support

COUNSELLING

A good counsellor can help you understand more about yourself and find strategies to help you cope with the loss of baby. Having some space and time to speak openly about how you feel without judgement or criticism can make a huge difference too.

Research suggests that it does not really matter what type of counselling you choose. It is more important that you trust and respect your counsellor and that you feel there is a good 'fit' between you. While it can help to find someone with experience of working with pregnancy loss, it should not be essential. Any good counsellor should be able to help you. If you feel that they do not 'get it', tell them and explain why. It may be that your counsellor has not got experience in working with pregnancy loss, but can work very well with other difficult feelings like anxiety and low mood. If you really do not feel comfortable, even after explaining things, it is best to end the sessions and find someone else. This can prove difficult to pluck up the courage, but it is worth it.

If you are seeking counselling on relationship and, or, sexual problems during this time, then find a couples counsellor.

If you are worried that you or your partner are having problems coping with grief, you may need further treatment and counselling. There are support groups that can provide or arrange counselling for people who have been affected.

Please go to our website (www.angelwingsgifts.co.uk) and subscribe to receive information on our support page on all local and national services.

References

Engel, George (1959). "Is Grief a Disease? A Challenge for Medical Research" in *Psychosomatic Medicine,* Lippincott, Williams & Wilkins

Ross and Kessler (2005). On Grief and Grieving, Scribner

Journal

Printed in Great Britain
by Amazon